- A Yoga Journey -
HEART ROOTED IN SKY

Sarah Pierroz

Library and Archives Canada Cataloguing in Publication

Title: Heart rooted in sky : a yoga journey / by Sarah Pierroz

Names: Pierroz, Sarah, author.

Description: Poems.

Identifiers: Canadiana (print) 20220160015 | Canadiana (ebook) 2022016004X | ISBN 9781771616089 (softcover) | ISBN 9781771616096 (PDF) | ISBN 9781771616102 (EPUB) | ISBN 9781771616119 (Kindle)

Classification: LCC PS8631.147555 H43 2022 | DDC C811/.6-dc23

Published by Mosaic Press, Oakville, Ontario, Canada, 2022

MOSAIC PRESS Publishers
www.mosaicpress.ca
Copyright owner ©SarahPierroz2022

Printed and bound in Canada

ONTARIO ARTS COUNCIL
CONSEIL DES ARTS L'ONTARIO

an Ontario Government agency
un organsime du gouvernement de l'Ontario

Funded by the Government of Canada
Financé par le gouvernement du Canada

Canadä

ONTARIO
CREATES

MOSAIC PRESS
1252 Speers Road, Units 1 & 2, Oakville, Ontario, L6L 5N9
(905) 825-2130 | info@mosaic-press.com | www.mosaicpress.ca

- A Yoga Journey -

HEART ROOTED IN SKY

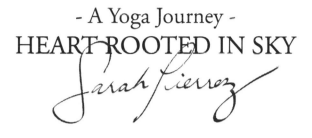

For those who dare to drop their armour

REVIEW
Heart Rooted In Sky, by Sarah Pierroz

"Sarah Pierroz's *Heart Rooted in Sky* reveals the direct experience of the body, mind, and the natural world as vibrantly joyous.

We are taken on an intense journey deep into the body and the mind, back and forth on an existential pendulum of fear and beauty.

With both poetry and illustration it makes us open our hearts like the sky to each other and all of life. This book is one to sit with and come back to like a friend so that its insights sink in through words, imagery and the imagination."

(- Richard Freeman, Yoga Teacher and Scholar)

BIOGRAPHY

Sarah Pierroz is a Canadian artist and international arts educator. She studied the integrated Arts & Science Program at McMaster University, then specialized in 'Artist in the Community' Education at Queen's University, both in Canada.

For over 15 years, she helped schools evolve in arts education in Africa, the Middle East, and Italy. She is now based in Thailand.

Along the way, Sarah studied and taught meditation, breath, and yoga techniques and textual studies in various cultures, such as: Tibetan Buddhism as it has migrated to India, Theravāda Buddhism in the forests of Thailand, Animism in flowing through the landscape of Bali, mystic poetry from Sufism, Tantric texts from wandering yogis in the Himalayas, living Vedic fire traditions, and ancient Sanskrit texts on yoga out of India.

Curious about different yoga and meditation practices, she learned from sincere monks in Thailand, pranāyāma (breathwork) masters in India, Tibetan practitioners in India and Nepal, and Zen masters and meditators in Bodh Gaya.

She holds specialized training in pranāyāma at the Kaivalyadhama Yoga Institute, in Lonavla, India. She is also an experienced Yoga Alliance teacher and taught immersive yoga and meditation for many years in Thailand and India. Sarah further integrates the meditative aspects of the breath into the practice of freediving, which she pursues with fondness and passion.

The quest for peace and its subsequent journey into fear compels her to continually explore the breath, heart, and mind.

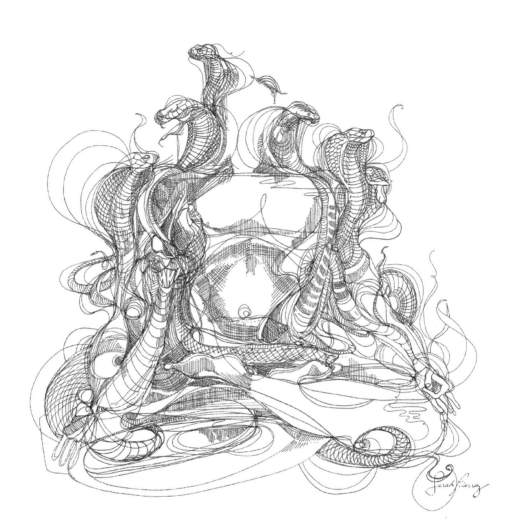

INTRODUCTION
What is Yoga?

When I was asked to write a book about yoga, I must admit that I struggled as there is much more to it than its popularized, influencer portrayal.

The modern image that springs to mind involves people in tights, configured rather precariously, on rubber yoga mats. But this is far from what I've come to understand yoga to embody.

Yoga has little to do with the extreme contortionist-like poses that we see presented in the media. If that were true, then decorated Olympians would hold the keys to enlightenment.

At its essence, yoga is a tool to explore our minds and connect with our deep inner nature.

There are numerous definitions of yoga and texts dedicated to its practice. Even so, a long history of translation and semantics can perplex the most committed among us.

Different schools of yoga offer conflicting views on what the experience of yoga is, or ought to be:

Is it a journey of service and devotion as found in Bhakti Yoga? Or a journey of self-inquiry and belief investigation as found in Jñāna Yoga? Or the path of forceful effort, as described in Hatha Yoga?

And yet, in this multiplicity of definitions, one does not triumph over the other. They all hold true.

The idea is that you set out on a path that helps you unravel and explore the aspects of your being that you would not normally encounter.

The gateway to a deeper sense of clarity and wisdom is through the parts of yourself that you tend to avoid.

Moving through different postures or the "āsana" component of yoga can get you to the doorway, but yoga itself is a personal inquiry.

Perhaps this is why the earliest documented yoga postures were typically seated positions, suitable for longer periods of meditation.

The physical body is considered one tool we have at hand to look more deeply within ourselves and into the nature of reality.

Practicing the physical discipline of yoga can help you see parts of yourself and of life that you may not otherwise have noticed.

For example, someone might overlook meditation because they can't be with their fiery side. They don't like to look at their chaotic, frustrated, lonely, sad, or uncomfortable states of mind.

Others might lack a sense of caring, compassion, or self-awareness, and overlook the effect of their yoga practice on their own body or how their actions impact others.

They might push themselves to do challenging postures or attempt positions that cause their body a great deal of pain and anguish.

Still, another might overlook a practice that tends to the body and its subtle internal techniques because they think that everything we experience has to do with the mind alone.

They might cut themselves off from the full spectrum of physical and emotional aspects that arise with a consistent and developed yoga practice.

A strong yoga practice will not only impact how you experience your life but also your relationships with others.

These relationships have the most powerful emotional influence on the body and mind that we encounter. They can challenge us to be more noble, truthful, and responsible for what we say and do.

Looking more consistently at your inner experience, along with how you relate to the world around you, can open the door to self-reflection.

The more you understand what you are fundamentally capable of experiencing and responding to, the stronger you become in your ability to truly experience the interconnectedness of all things.

A common translation that you might hear for the word "yoga" comes from the Sanskrit root "yuj" which relates to the concept of "union" or "yoking" a horse to a cart.

When your cart is connected to a horse, you experience the world much differently than when you are unhitched, alone, and feeling separate from everything else around you.

But at its heart, the path of yoga is a path of transformation.

It is considered a release from the state of delusion, or "avidyā" that we find ourselves in. We might perceive and understand reality to be far different from what it is. The antidote to this predicament is the development of clear thinking and wisdom.

As we apply wisdom and investigate our behaviours, beliefs, thoughts, and emotional responses, the outcome of yoga is experiencing an altered state of consciousness.

You come to experience who you truly are.

You come to experience life as it is.

This definition of yoga may seem utterly confusing. Aren't you always experiencing life as yourself?

Yes, but how is that experience for you?

Is there any pain or suffering tied up with that? How do you move through feelings of dissatisfaction, loathing, and discomfort? And how do you embrace experiences of pleasure and joy and love?

The path of yoga is a path through the pain, fear, anguish, and suffering that we prefer to avoid.

When we can make into our darkest moments with courage and strength, we come to experience a new understanding of life, where these things can no longer afflict us so deeply.

A metaphor that comes to mind is to think of yourself outside a burning building. Now imagine a small child is inside and you have to get her out.

You try to run into the building, but the intensity of the heat makes your skin feel like it's melting, you can't stop coughing from the smoke, your heart races, you can't see, you are acting from a place full of fear and doubt.

The experience becomes too much to handle and you have to run from the building.

Now, imagine yourself outside the same building, but you are trained in fire-fighting.

You've exposed yourself to extreme heat intermittently, in small doses. You've learned how to navigate rooms filled with smoke, and you've seen how fire sometimes behaves. You have the right gear on. You know how to handle high-stress situations.

You are not distracted by the sounds of anguish. And you've trained your mind to respond in high-performance mode, amidst the utter chaos around you.

So how do you experience that same fire? Differently.

You can enter the building, navigate the space, orient yourself, and deal with the conditions that confront you so you can find the child, and get her, and yourself, out of the building.

Similarly, yoga is a training tool, for your mind and perception of reality.

Yoga allows you to experience the same situation as anyone else but helps you not to suffer the distractions from what's happening in the very moment you find yourself in.

Yoga can be used to experience each moment as it truly is, with an open and courageous heart, if we so choose to embrace it head on.

ART, YOGA & NATURE

For me, creating art is like finding and revealing a secret little language.

When I was very young, I used to hide my drawings.

I would draw underneath tabletops, inside closets on the back walls, and on the linings of drawers. I knew I was talking with something bigger than me but kept the conversation extremely private.

When you make art, you find a small part of yourself, a little river inside. You ask a question, tap into it, and let it pour out from your fingers.

Sometimes the response comes from a painful moment, a violent gash to the veins. And you want it to be over quickly, but you swim in it instead.

Other times it flows from the quiet, deep ocean of the heart. It rises to you and overflows. You let it be as it is.

Making art is a way of listening to something beautiful passing through you, something beyond words. And it tends to be gone before you like.

I find these moments when I walk in the woods after heavy rain. My thoughts dissipate into the fresh air, fall into the gushing river, or crawl into the shadows of broad ferns hugging the ground.

The plants and natural world breathe a tenderness into me; I return from the path a little less bothered and a little more clear.

Walking can feel a lot like drawing.

When I first started practicing yoga, I felt the same. Over time, my body, breath, and mind started unraveling.

I began to release more stress, hesitation, fear, and doubt.

I learned how to watch myself from the outside, chiseling away the hardness and resistance to what was happening at that moment.

Whether in a meditative practice or by using specific, dynamic movements, there was a simple feeling of opening and a process of humble inquiry.

Once, I was adjusting a student in yoga class. She was in a deep, chest-opening posture called Uṣṭrāsana, or 'Camel posture.'

She said that in that posture, she felt a garden of flowers bursting from her heart.

I related and felt that feeling with her. I knew it from my practice. I could see it when she described it.

That night, I drew it and showed it to her. "Yes," she said, "this is it."

So I keep at it; I look for more connections between these wordless spaces of art, yoga, and nature.

"Tug on anything at all and you'll find
it connected to everything else in the universe."

(- John Muir, Naturalist and Environmental Advocate)

THIS STORY: ONCE UPON A TIME

This story of yoga is a little poem.

It describes a woman standing at the trailhead of a dark woodland passage.

It is the darkest path she can see.
It is a path that many avoid.

She journeys deeper into the forest and starts to feel a within. She feels different, more raw, vulnerable and open. She starts to look around and within and asks herself, "What is really here?"

Then, something odd happens. A tiny bird visits the woman. It lands on her chest and tugs at the thread holding her body and heart and 'everything else' together.

Out of this new space, she sprouts a little shoot. She grows into new limbs and becomes a part of the grand tree of life, eventually tasting the very fruit that it bears.

Or, more practically speaking, this is a story of a woman who goes on a journey of inner inquiry. She investiagtes her body, breath, and thoughts, and imagines another way of being.

By deepeing her understanding, she sheds her habitual behaviours, stories, and sense of identity. She continues on and transforms and opens to life as it unfolds.

No longer separate from the world around her, the woman lets go of her perception of reality to experience everything just as it is. She is able to connect more deeply with the world around her.

Sometimes the very place we fear to go is exactly the point where we must begin.

At its essence, this is a story of yoga, for it is a story of transformation, from the place of fear to space of love.

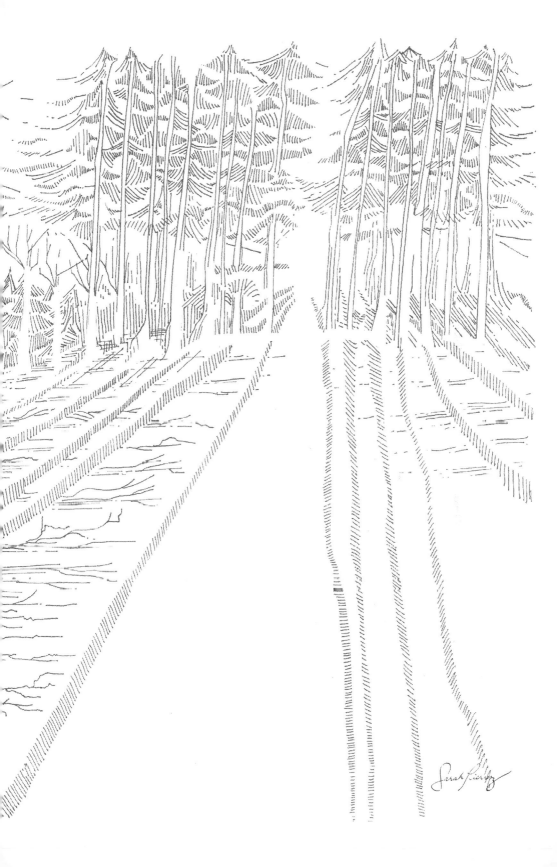

Outside,
at the edge
of a dense pine forest
of a sharp, dark,
but gleaming woods,
the local villagers tell stories
of many frightful risks.

They warn visitors,
of a biting, cold wind,
and slashing rains,
and sudden claps
of deafening thunder,
and flashes of disjointed lightning,
that vicious storms that rip through
the toughest of trees
and turn the world around it
into a burst of red flames.

Their voices drop
down low
and
their eyes dilate wider
when they speak of
of wild monsters,
and of unimaginable
wickedness
causing havoc
in the neighbouring
forest.

They hatch tales of
coy dogs
with insatiable appetites,
of musk deer with
razor-sharp fangs,
lurking,
and of unruly bears
stalking corridors,
hungry,
for some
sweetness.

The villagers serve breakfast
with stories of vicious snakes
that drop down from trees,
and constrict
unsuspecting hikers below,
until they feel the last heartbeat.

They detail the deadliest little
armoured scorpions
with venomous stings

and list all the other
dreadful creatures,
that particularly like
to devour unsuspecting females,
fresh from the city.

Ragged and weary,
the villagers
keep their stories
at their lips
and
close to their hearts.

They never wander far.
They stay close to home,
where they are learning
to make a fire
bright enough
to keep their
fears low.

The villagers spend all day
turning their mud-wall homes
into thicker concrete.
They build their walls
up higher,
and run long wires
across the valley
and raise up
bright strings of lights,
that stay on all night.

They import bigger screens
from the city
to get lost in titillating
Bollywood dreams.
They bump to beating drums
and blasting trumpets
and tiny high-pitched flutes
which shake the
entire valley floors.

Each villager is buzzing
on bottomless chai
and spoonfuls of jaggery.
When the night starts upon them,
they pop,
inject,
inhale
all sorts of powders and liquids.
They drink down
moonshine and homebrew.
They loosen up
in their tighter clothes.

[Whatever it takes, to endure it all.]

They fall asleep
only when
the sun starts to lighten the sky.
Only when they are certain
they will rise again.
With solemn faces,
with dead eyes,
they warn -
"Keep a far distance
from the darkness child."

What they really mean is -
"Go hungry."

I didn't pay these claustrophobic sounds attention.
I don't want them to win me over.

[Be savage.]
My heart called.
So, I stepped into
the open jaw
of the wolf,
into the darkest place
I could find.

I did not look back.

I am sure
I must appear a little mad
in the eyes of folks
who doesn't walk much?

I move on.

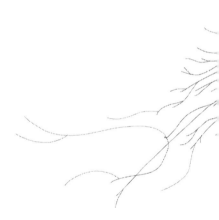

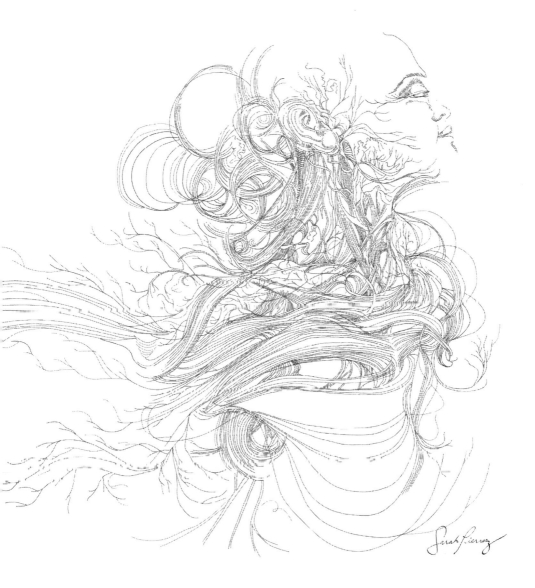

I walk down the path
leading to sun shadows
Towards
the sharpest mountain,
the coldest river,
the deepest water,
and to the bleached reef.
To the dried-up oasis,
and the thickly walled forest.
Towards the empty tundra.
Towards every fear.

I step into it.

I have no idea
where my foot will land.
I only know I have one foot
to touch down to earth
while the other lifts and rises,
to touch the sky.
And this is enough
to stand on.

Past fallen trees,
winding paths,
at the top of the hill,
amongst wavering fresh cedars,
and the bluest of old-growth evergreens,
past the rhododendrons bursting
asunder in red flames,
I find an unusual spreading sequoia
resting in ash-laden soil.
She is quite out of place.

Her bark is a warm, brown,
and strong,
and thick,
and furrowed,
and growing higher
than the mind could ever hope.

A soft breeze caresses her tallest,
most tender leaves.
Then it does the same
to my
skin.

I rest underneath her clearing.
The ground is soft after a morning rain,
Still cool and wet,
my feet sink in
slowly
and feel skinny blades of grass
in between my toes,
down to the soft moss,
which blankets my body from underneath.

It's an enchantment to pause.

White hills, white thighs,
happily, nakedly, exposed
on a
bear path.

I let my hair down.
Golden rays of light
scatter through.
The light, the warmth
slowly play across my face,
feeling like the utmost
penetrating
kiss.

It's just that.
It's just like this.
There is the sun,
the breeze,
the silent space
above.
So simple, it frightens me.
So simple, it excites me.

The sky,
holds a moving city
of voluptuous cathedrals
of transparent stone
made from dissipating clouds.
It holds all the winged creatures, soaring:
the eagle, the finch, the dragonfly,
along with everything else
that eventually falls,
all the same.

I try to place my thoughts, my doubts,
my longings in this space,
but they are too heavy for the sky to hold.
It is a horizon that spreads out
needless fear, and unneccessary language.
It pulls consonants
so far apart
that insignificant vowels
drop
like fat molecules of rain
to the soft ground.

Words vanish

into
raw,
natural,
life.

Then suddenly,
a bird swoops in,
a blue magpie would be exact.
She lands on my chest
for a moment,
hops around lightly,
then perches on my clavicle.

I barely feel her little claws,
light like eyelashes.
She tilts her head
side-to-side
and, with one eye, penetrates
my deep eyes
of hopeful sorrow.

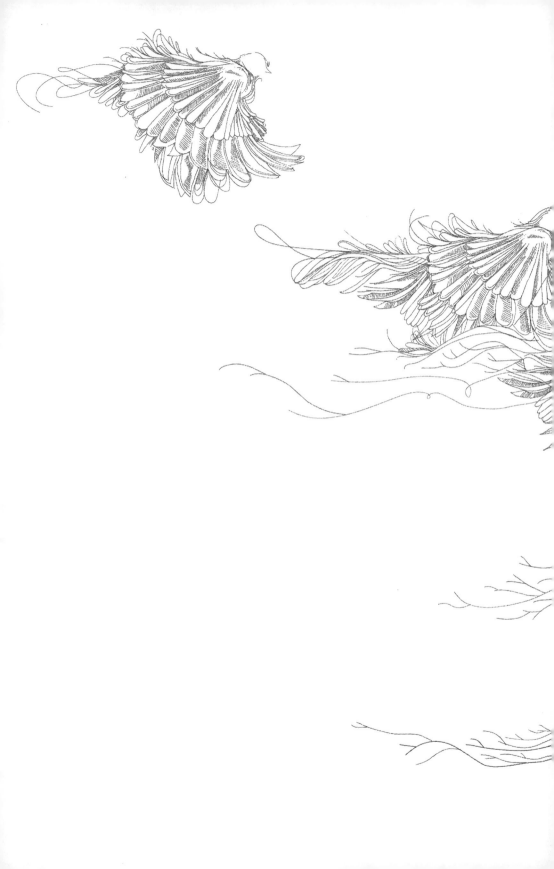

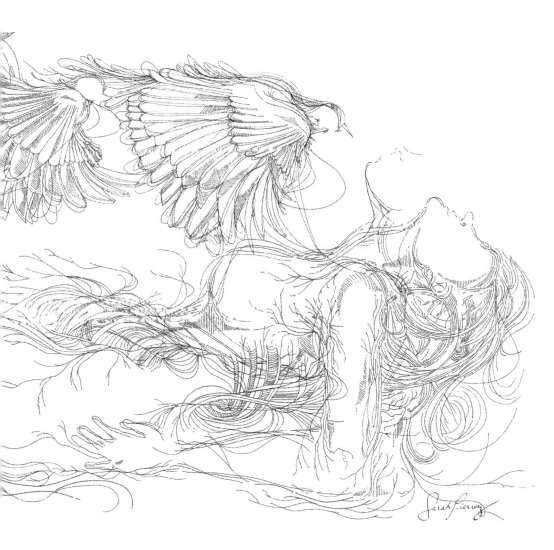

Then, the little magpie taps her beak down lightly.

Once.
She hits the bone
just underneath,
then digs her claws
in a little deeper
and braces herself
so she can knock harder,
this time rapidly,
as though to wake me up.

She is searching for seed.

My hands are empty.
My chest is empty.
I have already given up on patience,
on holding out sweet honey and sesame
waiting for you to come (back).

I don't flinch.
I pull a long silky,
deep breath in.

Then, when she finds the exact place,
just where the heart
grows hard with stories,
just where it parches up,
the little magpie
hammers
her little beak downward.
In one strong, exact blow,
she pierces through
my wonderfully rough bark
as a woodpecker might.

Inside this simple flesh,
at my navel,
the most beautiful place on earth,
where life began in a time before breath,
she takes hold of a fine,
messy golden thread.

She tugs at it swiftly, but slowly.
Careful not to break it.
I can feel the edges
scrape the sides of my skin.
Despite the discomfort,
I let her pull.

[Do not give nor resist, Little One.]

She waits until the golden thread
is completely released.
Then, she lets out
a little burst of song.

With each inhale,
my chest rises,
the bird digs more.
It starts to hurt.

[Never mind that, darling.]

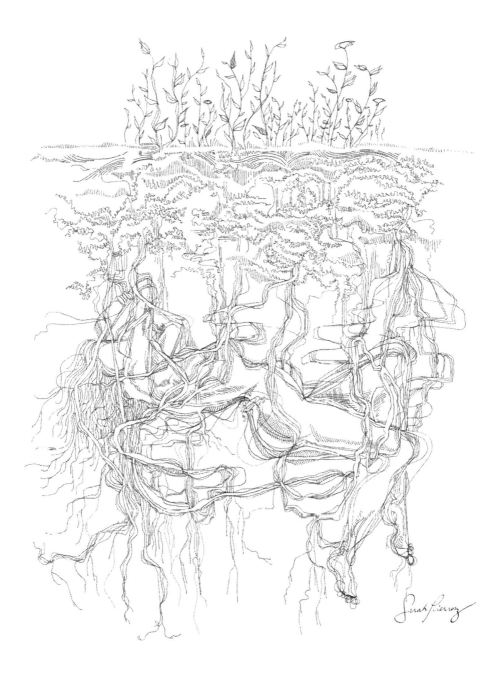

I start to unravel
and am made humble like dust and ashes.
A small nest of roots
now grows by the magpie's tiny claws.
Soon, a fresh shoot
begins to sprout out
from my belly.

I didn't want to look.

Every story I thought was mine,
is pulled out for me to see and question:
What is this really?

I look.
Her sleek, shining dark wings
glisten in the sun.

I wonder:
How did you get in?
and
How long will it be
until you leave?

I try to get up,
to ignore this small growth,
to ignore this invasive bird
and go about my walk.
But there isn't much to do.
There's isn't much to do at all.
She stays with me.
She has no shame.
This raucous little bird
is now perched on my shoulder.
She shakes her long tail feathers
up and down
proudly.

I sit.
She plucks more. Then again.
Pulling.
Snapping her head to the side
again and again.
Reaching.
Releasing.
Relentlessly perforating
Puncturing.
A growing fracture expands.
Memories that are so deeply forgotten come up,
through the fragile tunnel
right through this new PICC line.

I barely recognize myself.
Longer and thicker strands
buried along deep fascial lines,
twisted in the gut,
embedded in the ligaments,
all pull up.

She just continues to tear away.
[Turn over.]
There is always
another side.

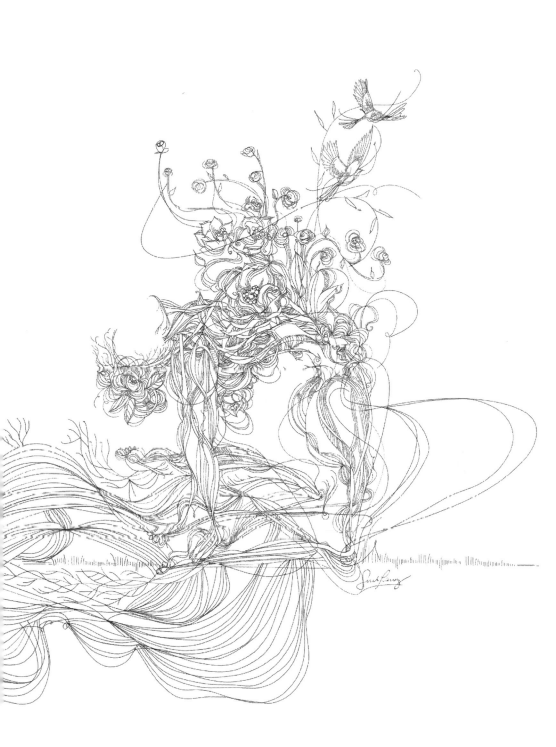

Now, when she pulls,
my fibres taut,
my joints bend.
Unfolding.
Expanding.
Contorting.
Cascading.
Unearthing.

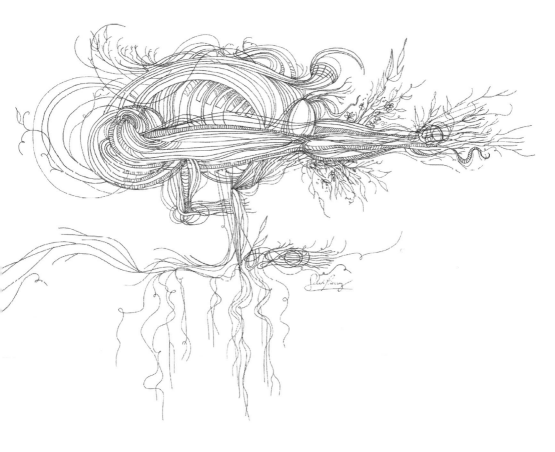

The more I expose and offer,
the less it hurts.
[Face it all the same.]

Now, all that is left
is what is,
naturally.
Here.

The sprout grows thicker.
It spirals up to the sky,
almost a small tree
in its own right.

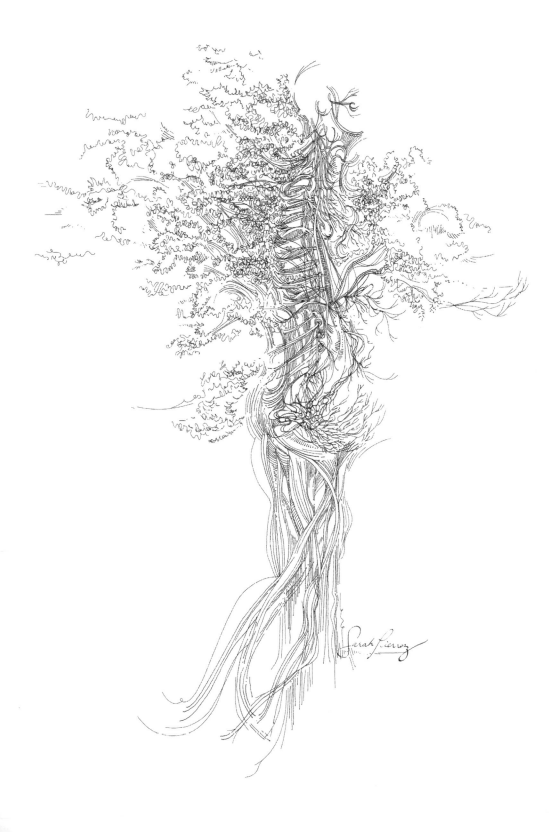

Everything deep inside my smile:
greed,
desire,
jealousy,
hatred.
All brew and boil,
wickedly,
to the surface.
The way you used to look at her,
the way you left me and took the castle.
The way the ground pulled from under my feet.
The day when everything I knew was obliterated
The day a stone grew into my heart.
The way I wanted you dead too.

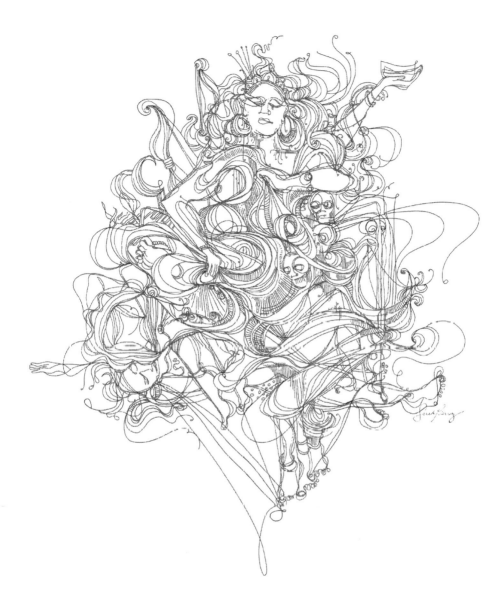

I didn't want [you] to see that.

Beasts and merciless thoughts,
and dormant raging dragons,
and wholly unsayable inclinations,
creep up the bark, slowly.
They clot and curdle,
then pour out
like a thick syrupy resin
along my trunk.
"Hold us closer!" they beg,
"Pull us back in!"
"Make us a part of you!"
"Don't forget!."

[Inquire.]
[Is that really True?]
[Is that really You?]

What have I brought into the forest?
These dark shapes,
Although I have met some before,
in others,
in our conversations,
in our happenings.
I never let them out
to roam so freely.
I avoided the portal they opened.
I now watch how they stir my suffering.

The sun goes down.
I rise to my feet and stand on the tips of my toes.
But my heels fall flat in protest.
With so much more space,
very little stands on them.

I feel like I can't go on
without my stories.

[Exactly.]
{Question them.}

No longer perfectly proportioned,
my fingertips reach as tall as the Himalayan peaks.
I twist.
A synovial hinge joint straightens here and there.
My legs become thick roots.
They cut down further
into weathering rock,
and search mossy plains for water.
A flicker of optimism
lifts my chest.

Things are as they are.
And they are not mine.
They are not me.

I offer all this space
to something else,
to something more.

Now,
I am ready.

Now,
I can offer seed.

The tree grows taller,
climbing for light.
My arms are thickened branches.
Life-lines extend from my palms.
Strands of copper-coloured fibres
jet out at all angles,
and birds fly through and in between them.

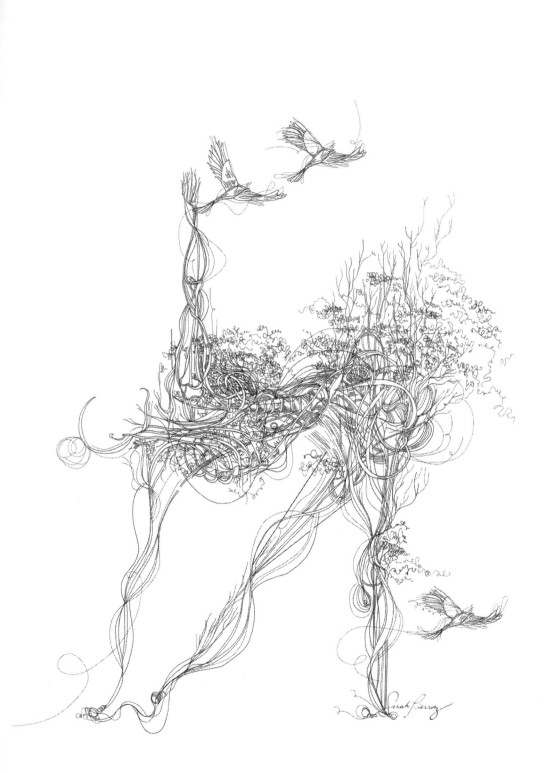

I feel you with me again;
I can no longer feel difference.
This tree - my veins
My fingers - your fingers
My roots - your roots

Our ribs stitch together
The breath passes through both our lungs.

[What a gift.]

But then, just like the exhale,
you are gone.

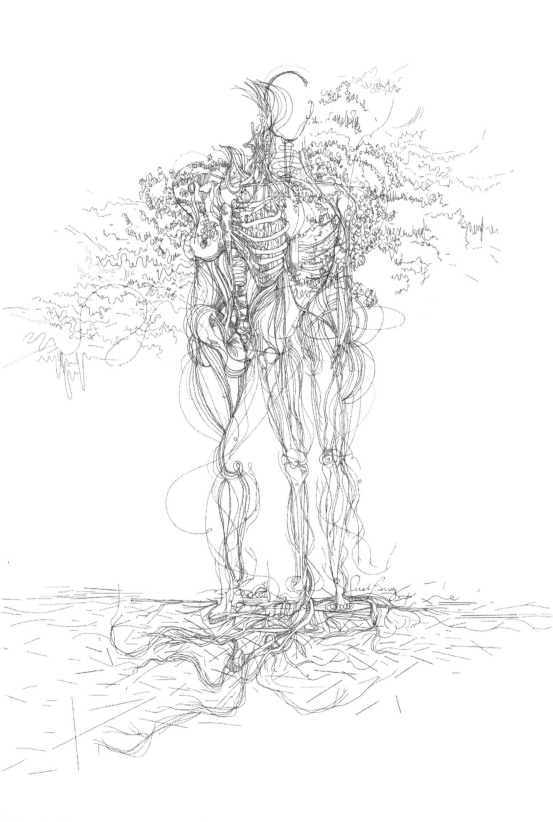

Alone,
I open into
A place to mourn, again
and hope
and wonder.
A place to open
to life,
to loneliness,
to noble failures,
to tragic chance,
to babies,
to death,
to ruins,
to bursts of joy,
to being blasted apart,
to being road rash on asphalt,
to a grain of dirt,
to the flowers that bloom out from it,
and to being food for jackals.

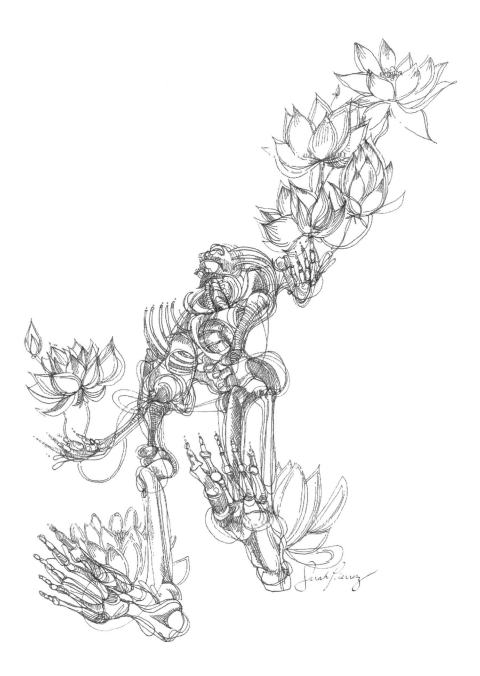

Nothing is mine to hold.
All that is inside me,
all that is dearly clinging,
all my secretly guarded possessions,
my pride,
my identity,
my endlessly unending addictive thoughts,
burst out like seeds,
from a tightly packed pine cone,
inside a cleansing fire.

A pulse
comes into my voice.
But all I can do is whisper,
sweetly,
one word,
pushed through hungering teeth,
'more.'

When in doubt,
increase the intensity.

[There is nowhere else to hide.]

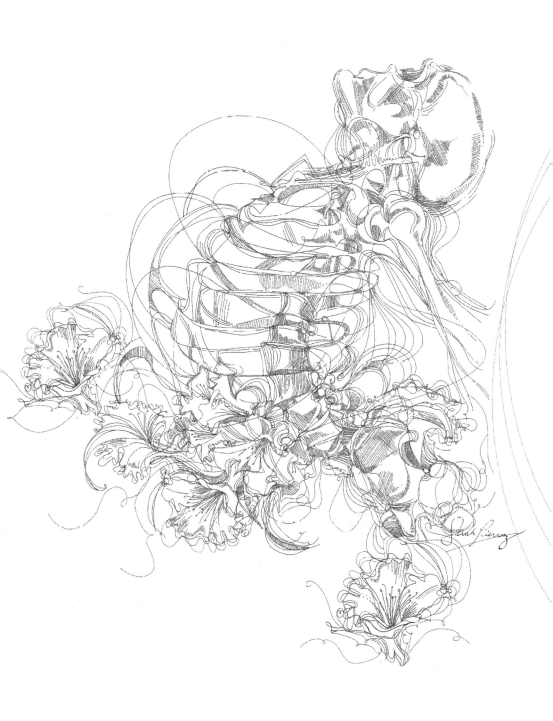

I find a deeper arch
in my lumbar,
more height in my breast,
branches rise higher and twist and curl,
sprinting their way towards the sun.
Little shudders move up
through my vertebrae,
growing space in between my ribs,
between all this flesh and bone
that life stitched together.
A serpent bellies around my trunk.
I take no notice.
It moves along its way.
[These things pass.]

Then, I raise my chest,
to help the little bird cut,
right through my heartwood,
right to the pith,
right to the pain,
until nothing is left,
not even detritus.

She is my carving tool.
She brings me to the sky.

Whatever was my foot
now pulls away from the earth.
I am light enough to stand with the clouds.
In the rain, the quickening sun,
my heart dissolves in the sky.
And at the same time,
it roots in the sky.
Nothing certain can reach me here.
If I had had other senses,
I am certain
there are other things
I would come to know.

Then, she snaps.
The body
falls,
glides,
back down
to the ground,
back down to the earth,
where parts can burn
and decompose and
cycle through again.

I am thirsty.
My veins
grasp further for water,
for its flash and gleam.
I let it drink me,
while feeling
its cool suppleness
and grace.

I am
in a place
unclaimed.

Open.
Tall.
Free.

The little magpie perches
on the nest of golden threads
at my feet
and offers a small white flower upon my head,
and one word to protect it.

[Truth]

This little shoot is now a place
to shelter newborn leaves below.
Where other small winged friends nest -
like red-bellied woodpeckers, crows,
cardinals, and sandhill cranes.
Where silkworms safely lay eggs.
Where small brown-bellied squirrels
chase each other with glee.
Each fingertip,
now ten small succulent mulberries,
growing wildly ripe and ever so sweet.

[You must look hard to see what is(n't) there.]

My heart
needs (no) more.

The little magpie serenades me
with the forgotten song of the wanderer:

It is as simple as this.
In this changing field,
wear your skin lightly.
Just experience what is happening thought to thought.
There is no need to hold on to any one.

To feel the earth.
[Be the breeze]
To feel the mountain.
[Be the soft mist]
To enter the fire.
[Be the fuel]
To enter the sky.
[Unravel. Dissolve.]

Don't let the language interrupt you.
Feel the vibrancy of it all.
Don't fall into fiction.

Smile at the lament of old, scared ones.
Leave their stories for the children.
Leave your stories for the compost.
Listen to the timeless tales of wisdom inside instead.

Then she is gone.

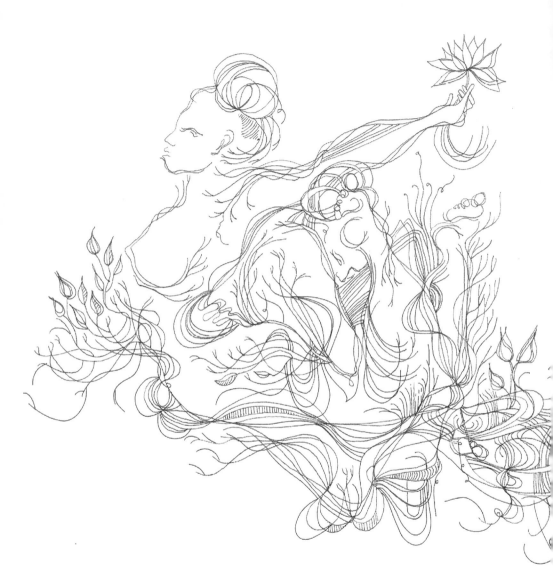

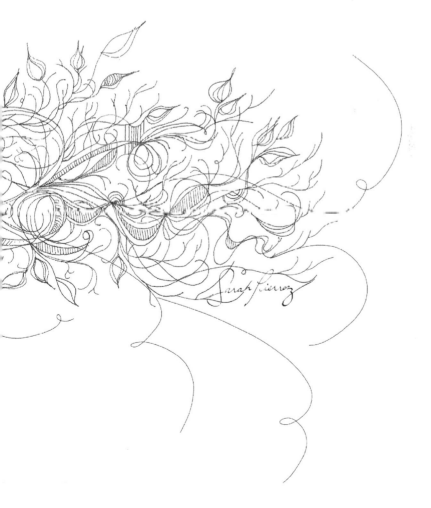

Her message
stays in my veins:

Life
isn't meant to be handed over to the wind,
and you aren't meant to bend
and break at every sway.

Instead, be the sky.
You.
Cloudless woman.

Be Open. Fearless.

Love.

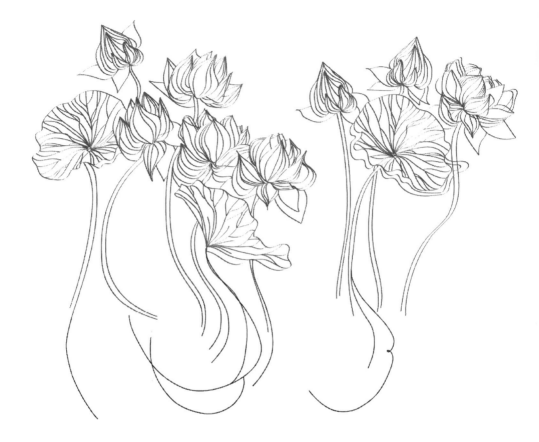